Colorectal Cancer
A True Story

K. Raveendran

DEDICATION

To my beloved wife (Late) K. Prasanna

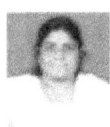

TABLE OF CONTENTS

1 Introduction

Just the mention of the word Cancer creates a tremor through your body. A feeling of chillness on your spine. Every year, millions of people are affected by the dreaded disease in one form or other. The major types of cancers are breast cancer, liver cancer, lung cancer, leukemia (blood cancer), prostate cancer, colon cancer (also known as bowel cancer), rectal cancer, skin cancer, and cervical cancer.

In fact, people are clueless about the cause of cancer. How fast it spreads and how it affects the health of the person afflicted with any form of cancer?

Though the exact cause of cancer is unknown, the unusual growth of cells called, gene mutation, causes cancer. In certain cases, use of some drugs like oral contraceptives, hormonal drugs used in the treatment of osteoporosis, and frequent abortions, may trigger cancer cells.

In addition, use tobacco in all forms including smoking is the largest cause of cancer, especially lung and mouth cancer, which is over 35% of the total cancer patients in the world.

Further, vitamin D deficiency, especially amongst women confined to home, causes spread of cancer.

I take this opportunity to bring forth a comprehensive experience for the benefit of patients, their family, friends, relatives, or anyone who is interested to know more about bowel/colon/rectal cancer.

Unlike any other form of disease, cancer not only ruins the person affected, but also his/her family's financial conditions as the cost of cancer treatment is very high. The treatments especially chemotherapy and radiation therapy costs much higher than the cost of surgery.

Therefore, it is very important to know about various forms of cancer, its symptoms, diagnosis, and treatment, diet requirements and planning.

As the adage goes, if detected early, the disease i.e. any form of cancer can be cured. Otherwise, it is extremely difficult to cure the disease as there are limited options and medication available as of now. However, in some cases, the disease can be controlled, but cannot be cured.

The following information is not a fiction or imagination. This is the real story of my wife Prasanna, diagnosed with rectal cancer in September 2010.

I am not a doctor, but gained in-depth knowledge about the disease during the course of treatment of my wife, spread over 26 months from September 2010 until January 9, 2013.

There are instances in which the physician or surgeon will not tell you the whole truth, sometimes ignore patient concerns, and do what they like.

It is, therefore, essential to know more about the treatment, its side effects, and what needs to be done especially in the last stages of the patient, i.e. **palliative care.**

The main purpose of this book is to help rectal, colon or colorectal cancer patients, their family, friends and relatives, or those who do not have any knowledge of the disease and do not know how to proceed with the diagnosis, treatment, and patient care during the aftermath of positive diagnosis.

It also tries to emphasis the need for proper palliative care of the patient, especially during the last stages, i.e. during the remaining few months of his/her life.

It is very painful, sometimes extremely sad, helpless and above all, living a life of wretchedness. However, all hope is not lost since the diagnosis and treatment over the past over two decades has brought in new technology, medicines, diagnosis techniques, improved treatment regimes and palliative care.

You may come across many instances of doctors not giving proper advice and sometimes neglect in treatment.

Therefore, my aim is to help patients and their immediate family members by providing helpful information and need for caution during and after the treatment. This will come in handy during difficult situations.

2 Diagnosis

As already mentioned in the introduction, this is the real story of a female rectal cancer patient i.e. my wife, Prasanna, aged 48 years. Like any other human being, she was happily married, have a loving husband and a lovely daughter. Things were all smooth, life was comfortable, no worries about future.

However, during the past few years everything was abnormal. A few health problems started appearing from nowhere. In the beginning, problems like fever, tiredness, a little weight gain etc. were noticed. However, we thought it may be due the onset of diabetes, or BP. This was sometime in the year 2007.

A thorough check up was done in a corporate hospital, conducting all the necessary tests. The reports indicated that she is having diabetes and high level of triglycerides.

Therefore, treatment started for diabetes and BP and after a year, she became normal and treatment continued for the same. However, we never thought about cancer.

In July 2010, while sitting on the sofa, she felt some wetness on the hip side and on inspection; she found that her panties were wet with some water like fluid.

She told about this to me and I thought it may be some discharge of fluids. However, both of us had no idea that this may be due to rectal cancer.

This incident was not pursued immediately with any medical examination. However, after two months of the first instance sometime in September 2010 one more incidence of watery fluid discharge noticed from rectal area.

This time, both of us decided to have the same brought to the notice of a good gastroenterologist and gone for medical opinion. After physical examination, the doctor suggested to do a Colonoscopy.

The next day a colonoscopy was done and the doctor and my wife were shocked to see that a big tumor of the size of 4 x 3 cm, about three cm from the anal verge. Here is an image of the Colonoscopy report.

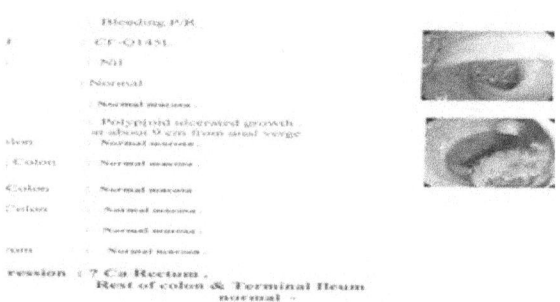

The doctor's face showed it all, as he did not believe that such a big tumor was there without giving any signals. Prasanna also felt very sad. However, she was a very brave women. She discussed the matter with the doctor along with me.

As per the advice of the gastroenterologist, we decided to go in for an immediate surgery for the removal of the tumor.

Following the colonoscopy test, a CT scan, and an Ultra Sound scan of the whole abdomen done and the tumor was re-confirmed.

Sometimes, certain incidents in life become an indicator of things which lies ahead like the following one. After diagnosing rectal cancer, we remembered about an incident that happened some four years back i.e. in the year 2006.

While travelling in a long distance train journey, a woman co-passenger told my wife that she is going to visit her daughter living in Noida, near Delhi and she underwent treatment for rectal cancer, and she fully recovered from the dreaded disease after treatment, and she thanked god for saving her life.

The women told that she felt something was wrong with her body, gone for a medical examination, and found to have rectal cancer. She advised my wife about the complication of treatment and asked her to be vigilant.

Normally, men are the victims of rectal cancer. However, women are also afflicted with colon or rectal cancer. In US alone more than one and a half lakhs people, both men and women, are diagnosed with rectal/colon cancer, each year.

In majority of cases, it is detected in advanced stages and therefore, loss of life is also high. Over 50000 patients die of rectal/colon cancer in the US alone, and you can imagine, worldwide, what will be the figure? It will be in several lakhs.

We never thought or imagined that my wife diagnosed with rectal cancer a few years later, as there were no symptoms to be doubtful.

Even there was no known history of any one in her family having rectal cancer. It is normally believed that cancer spreads through hereditary or from the same gene. In her case, it was not.

After thorough reading of various cancer related information on the web, specifically related to rectal cancer, I have learnt the following information, which is very crucial for cancer patients and his or her family.

This relates to diagnosis and treatment, various side effects of diagnosis techniques, radiation therapy, chemotherapy, medicinal side effects, and its remedies. Some of the important signs and symptoms of Colon/Rectal Cancer that you must observe for are:

1. Change in bowl habits like diarrhea, constipation, or narrowing of the stool.

2. Frequent feeling to have bowel movements.

3. Rectal bleeding, dark stools, **blood in the stool** *(this is a very important sign that you must take immediate medical opinion from a gastroenterologist or a medical oncologist).*

The bleeding may be due to hemorrhage, polyps, or tumor. Sometimes due to constipation, bleeding can occur, but should not ignore this particular symptom.

4.   Stomach pain, weakness, and fatigue, sometimes very frequent fever, and even weight loss, which may be due to colon or rectal cancer.

Screening tests for detection of colorectal cancer

Some of the tests advised by the physician to detect colorectal cancer or polyps are the Fecal Occult blood test, Fecal Immunochemical test, Stool DNA test, Sigmoidoscopy, Colonoscopy and/or CT scan.   Here is a small brief about these tests for your general information.

Fecal Occult Blood Test

The fecal occult blood test (FOBT) is done to find occult blood (blood that cannot be seen with the naked eye) in feces (stool).

The FOBT detects blood in the stool through a chemical reaction.   If this test is positive, a colonoscopy will be required to find the reason for the bleeding.

Although cancers and polyps can cause blood in the stool, other causes of bleeding can occur, such as ulcers, hemorrhoids, diverticulosis (tiny pouches that form at weak spots in the colon wall), or inflammatory bowel disease (IBD or colitis). This test can be done at home itself and need repeated tests, normally every year.

Fecal Immunochemical Test

The fecal immunochemical test (FIT), also called an immunochemical fecal occult blood test (iFOBT), is a newer kind of test that also detects occult (hidden) blood in the stool. This test reacts to part of the human hemoglobin protein, found in red blood cells.

Sigmoidoscopy

Sigmoidoscope is a small video camera i.e. about 2 feet length, used to examine the inner part of rectum and partial area of the colon.

Here is an image of a Sigmoidoscope.

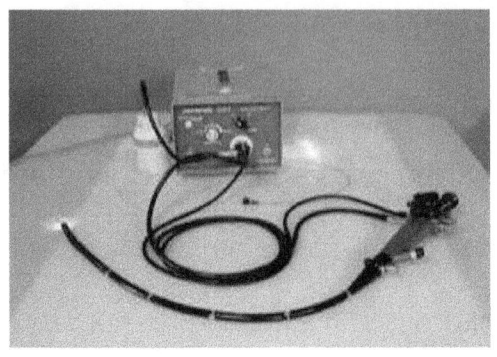

Courtesy: www.trialx.com

However, for a full examination of the colon, the doctor uses a Colonoscope, which is much larger than a Sigmoidoscope and fitted with video camera.

Here is an image of a Colonoscope.

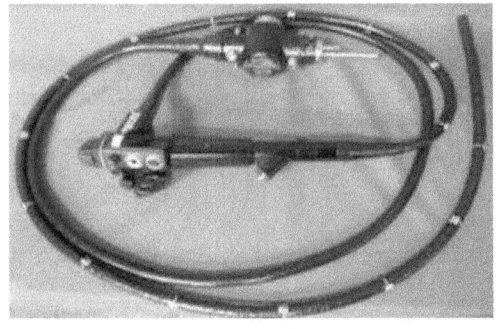

Courtesy: www.kewinmd.com

You may visit sites like www.cancer.org (by American Cancer Society) for detailed information about these tests and its side effects, if any.

Another test that doctors normally recommend for identifying colorectal cancer is the DCBE (Double Contrast Barium Enema) test, which is like an X-ray test.

However, a colonoscopy test will give better picture and more accurate results. You can check with your doctor for detailed information and to find out which the best is for you.

Virtual Colonoscopy/Whole Abdominal CT scan

The CT scan gives more accurate images than the colonoscopy as it takes several images and gives a combined result.

Genetic (DNA) Risk Analysis

The latest advancement in the diagnosis and treatment of cancer, of all types, is the use of hereditary gene risk analysis tests.

There are various types of gene (DNA) analysis and testing services available across the globe. Some of the most advanced screening tests using DNA (gene) are as follows.

Breast, Ovarian & Endometrial Cancer (known as women cancers)

ATM	EPCAM	CHEK 2	BRCA 1
BARD 1	RAD 50	CDH 1	BRCA 2
BRIP 1	RAD 51 C	TP 53	PMS 2
MRE 11 A	PALB 2	PTEN	MSH 6
NBN	STK 11	MUYTH	MLH 1
			MSH 2

Colorectal Cancer

BARD 1	EPCAM	CHEK 2	BRCA 1
BRIP 1	RAD 50	CDH 1	BRCA 2
MRE11A	RAD51C	TP 53	PMS 1
NBN	PALB 2	PTEN	PMS 2
SMAD 4	STK 11	MUYTH	MSH 6
APC	MLH 3	AXIN 2	MLH1
BMPR1A	TSC 1	TSC 2	MSH 2

Prostate Cancer

ELAC 2	EHBP 1	HSD3B2
MSMB	RNASEL	HSD17 B3
BRCA 2	SRD5A2	PTEN
HPC 5	KA 11 (CD 82)	CHEK 2

Another important test for identification of cancer causing gene is the analysis of genomic profile of a tumor/leukemia to identify the mutations in genes like K-RAS, EGFR, BRAF, and HLA.

Further, a Pharmacogenetics Assay can help the doctor plan a most cost effective and more suitable medication based on the genetic architecture of the patient. This method can eliminate injurious outcomes and make therapy more effective.

Therefore, it is essential to talk about this with your medical oncologist and plan the treatment accordingly so that no money, time and efforts are wasted and the patient gets the best treatment.

Sometimes, depending upon the patient's condition, the doctor may not wait for these tests, but straight away, based on his experience, start appropriate treatments.

Here is a list of some of the best-known cancer gene testing labs.

You may ask your medical oncologist about the availability of this facility in the hospital. If not available, ask for the best places they have contacts or suggestions to arrange for the test.

In USA

www.labcorp.com

www.bcm.edu

www.foxchasecancercentre.org

www.genedx.com

European Union

https://www.myriad.com

India

ACTREC, Navi Mumbai - Research and Training arm of Tata Memorial Hospital.

1. www.actrec.gov.in

2. www.datarpgx.in (Datar Genetics Ltd., Mumbai)

Financial Assistance

Many patients are facing financial constraints for undertaking better and timely treatment. They may be looking for some kind of help.

There are many voluntary organizations, government agencies, and charities, offering financial help for poor and needy patients.

Here is a list of organizations you may contact for help.

Cancer Financial Assistance Coalition is one such organization and their website **www.cancerfac.org** and **www.cancercare.org** is some of the places where you can find list of organizations helping needy patients in getting financial assistance.

Another good organization is the US government program called Medicaid. Their web site **www.medicaid.gov** will give required information about the program.

In addition, R.A. Bloch Cancer Foundation, website **www.bolchcancer.org** is a good place for getting more information about financial aid.

American Cancer Society, Cancer Survivor's Fund, Cancer Research Institute, Children's Cancer Research Fund, Lungevity Foundation, Susan G Koman for the Cure, Vineman Cancer Charities Fund, etc are places where you can get funding related information and help.

In the U.K. there are many charitable organizations providing help to needy patients. Some of the well-known names are Marie Curie Cancer Care, Macmillan Cancer Support, Cancer Research, U.K.

In addition, if you search on the internet, you can find many such organizations either near to you or within your state or country, which will provide detailed information about financial assistance for treatment.

3 Surgery

You can imagine the amount of tension, fear, and helplessness the patient going through at that point of time. Just one day before the appointed date for surgery, I got my wife Prasanna admitted to Apollo Hospitals, Hyderabad, India (this is the only group of hospitals in India, accredited with Joint Council International (JCI).

These are the times when family support and especially close family members presence and empathy is expected by the patient. The surgery for removal of tumor from rectal area is a very difficult task and it takes about 4-5 hours for completion of the operation through a general open surgery. In her case, this was an Ultra Low Anterior Resection (ULAR) of the rectum, because the space available for stapling was about 2.75 cm from the anal verge, which normally should be a minimum of about 3 cm from the anal verge.

The surgical oncologist assured us that nothing to worry and it will be a successful operation. Only problem was that since the space available at the rectal area is less than three centimeters, it would be very difficult for him to connect the colon and rectum using Staplers (this stapler is used for connecting the colon and rectum after removing the affected area).

Given below is a link to a web site where, you can see the Low Anastomosis of Colon to Rectum using the End-to-End **Surgical Stapler Technique** for connecting the colon and rectum after surgically removing the affected tumor part. Copy and paste the following link on your browser to see how the stapler is used in the surgery.

http://www.atlasofpelvicsurgery.com/7Colon/6LowAnastomosisofColonto
RectumUsingtheEnd-to-EndSurgicalStaplerTechnique/ chap7sec6.html

The surgery was successful and after 5 hours in the OT, shifted her to the recovery room. For another 4 hours, she was in the surgical recovery room, and when there was no complication, they shifted her to the room.

In case of complications after surgery, the patient may be shifted to an ICU. In about 9 days she became normal since she was quite healthy. While handing over the discharge note, the doctor advised her to come back after 45 days for further preventive treatment i.e. Adjuvant Chemotherapy and Radiation Therapy.

Note: One information the surgeon and the oncologist hidden from us was the biopsy report of the removed tumor, which indicated that 4/8 lymph nodes of the tumor was positive.

Though the surgeon gave us the biopsy report, he did not tell us about the seriousness or explain about the significance of the same.

This was very crucial and very important information; because that indicates there is danger of the tumor cells spreading to other parts of the body through blood, viz. liver, pancreas, kidneys, lungs, brain, skeletal systems and so on.

In my opinion, every patient's immediate relatives, viz. father, mother, husband, brother, or sister, as the case may be, must ask the surgeon as well as the physician in charge of the case, about this fact immediately after the surgery and especially before discharge from the hospital.

Grading of Cancer

After the surgical resection, a few pieces of the tumor was collected as samples for biopsy and send for analysis. Normally this will take about 4-5 days and after that the biopsy report will be prepared and given to you through the surgeon/oncologist. During the lab tests i.e. biopsy, they do the grading (Staging) of cancer. There are four stages viz. Stage I, II, III and IV. In my wife's case, she was at Stage-II after surgery.

Doctors uses the term **TNM** to measure the extent or spread of cancer. T = the primary tumor, N = lymph nodes and M = Metastasis. You can get more information about this from the web site **www.cancer.gov**

4 Chemotherapy & Radiation Therapy

In most cases, depending upon the severity of the case, the medical oncologist/ radiologist, use either chemotherapy or radiation therapy for prevention or recurrence of the tumor. Sometimes, a combination of chemotherapy and radiation therapy used in the treatment.

Chemotherapy

As the name indicates, chemotherapy is the use of chemicals (medicines) which are potent to kill cancerous cells. Some of the most popular chemotherapy medicines used in the treatment of colon/rectal cancer is as follows:

5Fu (Fluorouracil)

Irinotecan

Oxaliplatin

Capacitabine (Xeloda) tab/injection

Avastin (Becuzimab) - for targeted therapy

Leucovorin

Cetuximab (Erbitux) - for targeted therapy

Nupogen (for increasing the TLC and platelet level in the body after chemotherapy)

*A **Pharmacogenetics** (refers to the study of inherited differences (variation) in drug metabolism and response)* **Assay** *will give better treatment options, medication that suites the patient, and reduce side effects (Adverse Drug Reactions). Therefore, if time permits, and affordable, it is a good idea to do the test in consultation with your medical oncologist.*

Side Effects of Chemotherapy

Some of the main side effects of Chemotherapy include

Hair loss

Diarrhea

Bleeding

Pain

Appetite changes

Feeling weak and tired (fatigue)

Nausea and vomiting

Swelling

Nerve changes called Peripheral neuropathy i.e. numbness, tingling, burning or weak feeling in different parts of the body. Normally hands and feet are the most affected area. In my wife's case, this was the recurring problem during chemotherapy and thereafter until the end.

Vein Damages (Prolonged intravenous injections of chemo medicines result in damages to the main veins, especially, on the hands. In such a case, the doctor will recommend the use of the Central nerve or a chemo port.

The chemo port is a titanium disc with a self-healing diaphragm in the center and a catheter that goes into your artery.

Here is an image of a Chemo port. Click the image to enlarge.

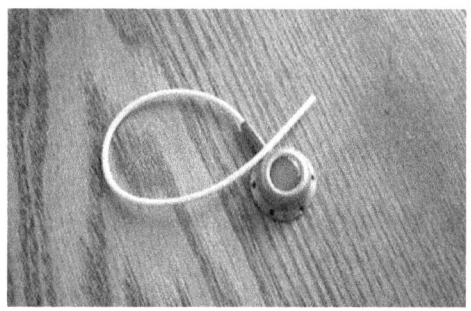

Courtesy www.cassera.net

In case you are curious to know more about the use of chemo port, you may visit the following web site at http://www.cassera.net/?p=27

Owing to continuous administration of chemo medicines for a long time, my wife's veins on both the hands, damaged. Owing to this, when she was in the MICU, doctors had to use her central vein i.e. the main vein on your neck for administering medicines, blood, and platelet.

Subsequently, during palliative chemotherapy and targeted therapy, they had to insert the chemo port on her right chest. This chemo port is very handy and can last for about 12 months.

Radiation Therapy

Radiation therapy is used for killing the cells surrounding the affected tumor area. Laser guided radiation is used for killing the tumor cells. There are external as well as internal methods used by the radiologist for treating the patient.

The different forms of radiation therapies are external beam therapy and internal beam therapy like branchy therapy. The most advanced radiation, external beam therapy is IGRT (image guided radiation therapy) technique, precisely targeted to the tumor cells at a 360° angle.

This technique is the most advanced and will cost you good amount. The next best is IMRT (Intensity modulated radiation therapy).

In certain case, you may not require the IGRT, instead an IMRT will give the same result and will save some amount of money. The differences between the two are very little, but cost wise, IGRT cost more.

However, please note that there are different techniques used by the oncologist/radiologist and based on the nature of disease, different kinds of equipments and treatment techniques are used.

Therefore, the doctor will be the right person to decide, which one will be the best for your patient. Normally there will be a group of doctors (a surgeon, radiologist, medical oncologist, and a physicist) in the treatment planning team.

Side effects of Radiation Therapy

The following are some of the main side effects of radiation therapy.

Extreme tiredness

Skin changes i.e. blackening of the surrounding area. Inflammation inside the mouth and throat.

When radiation is given in the pelvic area, it can affect the nerve system and curtail blood flow to the lower parts of the body like legs. However, the overall benefits of radiation therapy outweigh the side effects.

For more about radiation therapy, please visit the Government cancer web site at
http://www.cancer.gov/cancertopics/factsheet/Therapy/radiation

Special Diagnostic Tests

If anyone in the family is diagnosed with rectal/colon cancer, then a regular monitoring of Serum CEA (Carcinoma Embryonic Antigen) also known as CTC (circulating tumor cells) levels in blood on regular intervals, say in 2-3 moths period, during and after completion of treatment is a must. Any rise in the CEA level is an indication that the disease is spreading.

This is a very important aspect to be noted, because if there is a rising level of CEA/CTC in the blood, it indicates that the disease is spreading fast. Sometimes it cannot be controlled even with advanced chemotherapy. Therefore, make it a point to check the CEA level in blood periodically even during treatment. The physician may advice you not to do it frequently. However, my experience says that it is a good point to monitor the CEA level during chemotherapy at least once in 60 days or the least, once in three months.

It will be better to go in for a whole body PET-CT scan with contrast, most oncologists recommend this, and however, in certain cases only a CT or MRI is enough.

The PET-CT scan with contrast is very costly but it will give more accurate results. The cost of this test will be high, and varies from country to country, but worth it.

In India, it cost between Rs.33000-45000 i.e. about US $750. For more Information about PET-CT scan, contrast and its side effects, what precautions to taken before and after the test can be found at the following site **www.cancer.org**

After surgical removal of the rectal tumor, my wife was advised radiation therapy using chemo medicine Xeloda 500 mg x 2 (the technical name of the medicine is Capacitabine) and radiation @200 cGy/fr per day for 32 days.

Before starting the radiation therapy, a PET-CT scan with contrast or in certain cases, based on paying capacity and nature of the case, either a simple CT/MRI scan with contrast, will be done for marking radiation points i.e. for planning radiation.

Given below is an image of a PET-CT scan machine.

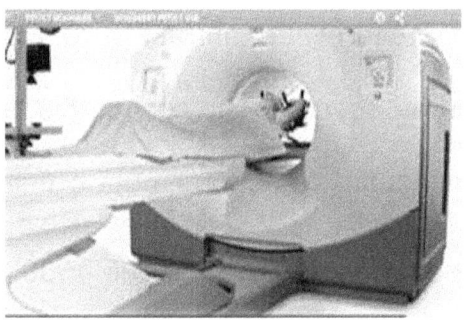

Courtesy www3.gehealthcare.com

We had chosen the IGRT method of radiation therapy and for this the PET-CT scan with contrast was done. The patient will be administered an intravenous injection using a radioactive substance (nuclear medicine) to identify the cancer affected cells for treatment planning.

There will be some complications like vomiting, loose motion, etc. However, normally there would not be many problems.

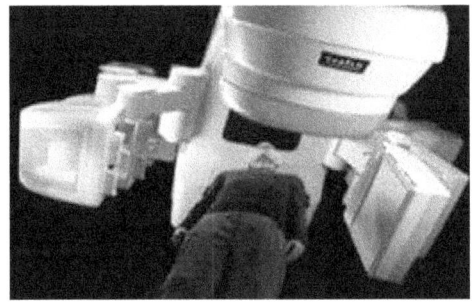

Image of a Radiation (IGRT) Machine.

Once the PET-CT scan is done, the next thing is the preparation of a mask based on the PET-CT report. This mask will be used during radiation for protecting the radiation area and its surroundings and to prevent any accidental damage to healthy cells, while administering the radiation doses.

During radiation treatment, the patient undergoes severe mental torture, burning sensation and sometimes severe pain. However, do not worry; the physician will prescribe preventive medicines for treating the side effects of radiation therapy.

The most essential thing needed for the patient is the emotional support from immediate family members. The patient has to drink lot of fluids (water or fruit drinks etc.) to control the heat in the body and eat nutritious food to ward off any side effects of the radiation.

In my wife's case, the problem started after a few days of radiation treatment. Severe burning (fire like) sensation on the rectal area with slight bleeding from the stapled colo-rectal area. Since stapling was used to connect the colon and rectum, the width of the jointed area of the rectum was reduced and there was difficulty in passing stool.

In addition, there was very little spasm. The surgeon told us that it would take some time to develop the spasm in the newly stapled rectal area. However, there was no improvement until the end, but passing stool was somehow manageable.

The situation was complicated because of the simultaneous use of Xeloda (Capacitabine) 500 mg x 2 tablets. This medicine causes loose motion as well as a burning sensation.

Very Important point to Note: The surgeon recommended adjuvant chemotherapy after the radiation therapy. However, he did not give specific instructions to the medical oncologist about the medicines to be used.

When complications developed later on, the surgeon told us that he meant using chemo medicines like 5Fu and other combination drugs along with radiation instead of the Xeloda 500 x 2 (1000 mg) tablets.

Please note the following point very carefully. Owing to the careless attitude or ignorance of the surgeon while advising the medical oncologist, he forgot to write instructions in clear terms like names of medicines, viz. tablets, or injections. As per the claims of the manufacturer of the Xeloda tablets (Roche) both the tablets and the injections give the same results. However, in our experience, the tablets did not give any visible benefits.

Many people who undergone chemotherapy indicated that injections gave better results. Cost wise there may not be much difference. Therefore, please check with your surgeon and medical oncologist about this point before starting treatment.

As much as possible, tell the surgeon to write the names of the medicines to be used in clear terms viz. whether injection or tablet, along with regular chemo medicines and radiation simultaneously, etc. so that it is very clear to the physician, what type of medicines and how it is to be used.

Another important aspect to remember is that in case the hospital where you take the treatment, if a two-in-one doctor i.e. if the medical oncologist and the radiologist is the same person, I strongly recommend to select two different doctors i.e. be the radiologist and medical oncologist separate.

The reason for this is that if the two-in-one doctor is very busy, there is greater possibility of the doctor making several mistakes, as has happened in my wife Prasanna's case.

He is quite capable and popular person, but being Director of the Cancer Institute, he handles chemotherapy and radiation therapy together; hence, his concentration will be much less, especially when the number of patients are more than he can handle.

Though there are few more medical oncologists in the hospital, the Director, who is a qualified medical oncologist as well as radiologist handle most of the cases with whatever left over for other medical oncologists to share.

The reason for this, I believe is, due to the amount of money he will be earning from so many cases.

In order to avoid this problem, check with the supporting staff or nurses in the chemotherapy section, to find out who is the best medical oncologist in their unit. From experience they know, who the best medical oncologist is.

If a doctor, who is of course, qualified as a radiologist and a medical oncologist, will sure to commit mistakes, especially if the doctor is having large number of patients. Therefore, in your own interest, please for god's sake as well as for your own sake; choose separate medical oncologist and radiation therapist for treatment.

Depending upon the nature of the case, the medical oncologist in consultation with the surgeon will decide what type of treatment to be given to the patient. In some instances the physician will start with chemo therapy first and radiation thereafter or vice versa.

In certain cases, they start the combined treatment with chemo medicines and radiation therapy together. This depends upon the severity of the case and patient's condition.

In my wife Prasanna's case, after the radiation treatment for 32 days @ 200 cGy/fr a day, she was advised to take rest for a month and then come back for the chemotherapy treatment.

During the rest period of 30 days, she had severe burning sensation in the rectal area, slight bleeding, and since her health was quite good, she managed somehow. Especially during nighttime, it was severe, particularly during cold wintertime.

The main problem with rectal cancer patients is the passing of stool, particularly when there is stapling or stitching between colon and rectum. Somehow, things were moving quite normally and were manageable.

Chemotherapy

After completing 32 days radiation therapy and taking rest for another 30 days, my wife, Prasanna was advised chemotherapy of 6 cycles. Each cycle is of 4 session's i.e. day 1-2 and after a gap of 14 days, day 3-4. Likewise, six cycles.

However, as a routine, lab tests like CBC (complete blood count) and Serum CEA was advised before the start of chemotherapy cycle. At this point of time, the CEA level indicated a sharp rise i.e. the count was 55, whereas before starting radiation, it was 2.6 (which is normal).

Both the doctor and we got worried about this revelation and he advised repeat of the CEA test. I even had gone to another well-known diagnostic centre to compare the test results.

Both the results i.e. the one from the hospital lab and the outside lab test of CEA has reconfirmed increase in the CEA level, which indicated that something is wrong somewhere.

Immediately, a whole body PET-CT scan was ordered by the radiologist and it brought the truth out. There was a 2.5 cm single lesion metastasis on the segment 2 of left lobe of Liver.

Imagine the amount of fear, tension, helplessness and frustration gone through by the patient. However, my wife was very brave and cool, though she asked me whether she will survive, because, already had a surgery, and radiation was done.

Then, came the news of a new secondary tumor in Liver. My wife as well as the radiologist, the surgeon, all got scared, because my wife was in Stage-II at the time of surgery. Now she is in Stage-III.

The surgeon and the radiologist-cum-medical oncologist had a quick discussion and decided to go in for the resection of the lever, because they felt this was the only thing that can ensure her survival.

They called me and asked for a quick decision from me. I also got scared and prayed god for the best. Then at night, I called the radiologist over phone and asked his personal opinion. He told me that there is nothing else, only the liver resection can save her. Luckily, the lesion was only a single one, though large.

Again, another great mistake the doctor/radiologist committed was that before the start of radiation therapy, he advised a PET-CT scan with contrast (whole abdomen) for marking the radiation points i.e. markings for treatment planning.

However, they should have advised to go in for a whole body scan with contrast, (cost wise, there is no extra amount to be paid) which could have given the exact condition of the patient including indication of any Metastasis elsewhere, since she had 4/8 lymph nodes positive at the time of surgery (LAR, low anterior resection). This may not be intentional, but definitely was a grave mistake.

This incident was in the first week of March 2011. On March 8, 2011 before the surgery, a whole abdomen Triphasic CT scan and Color Doppler was done to do the marking for the liver resection surgery.

The liver resection was done on March 9, 2011, which was successful and the surgical oncologist who had done the LAR earlier, shown me the piece of lever.

It was about a 4 cm square, and he told me that there is no spread of tumor anywhere in the left over liver. The liver will grow back into its normal size in about a month's time.

If you wish, you can have a look at the way, i.e. how liver resection is done. Just copy and paste the following web address onto your browser and place the cursor on the segmented parts (marked 1,2,3,......8, of liver to get an idea. Here is the link

http://www.hopkinsmedicine.org/liver_tumor_center/treatments/sur gery_remove_tumor.html

During or after the operation, there was no big problem and she was discharged after 9 days in the hospital. She was advised to report back after a rest of about 10 days for administering the adjuvant chemotherapy as planned earlier i.e. 6 cycles. The CEA level also has come down from 55 to 3.6, which was within the admissible range.

After the liver resection surgery, two pieces of the affected liver was sent for K-RAS mutation analysis by PCR. The K-RAS test repot shown that Sample (Exon 1), (Codons 12 and 13) has **No Mutation** also the 2nd sample (Exon 2), (Codon 61) also has **No Mutation.**

However, there was a small sentence in the middle part of the report, written in very small letter size that **"Sensitivity: 20% Mutant allele in the Wild-type allele".**

This was a crucial piece of information, which the doctor (radiologist-cum-medical oncologist) ignored. He had told me that since the mutation report is negative, i.e. No Mutation, there is no need to add any additional medicines to the chemotherapy.

I did not have any idea about this at that time. The graveness of this information came out after the completion of second cycle of chemotherapy.

Chemotherapy

The medication consisted of 5FU, Oxaliplatin and Leucovorin and the first and second cycle went very smoothly. However, on the 2nd leg of third cycle, she developed bleeding from rectal area. For this, they gave her some injections to prevent the bleeding and advised us to ignore the problem and continue with the remaining cycles of chemotherapy. However, the problem of bleeding from the rectal area continued.

When I gone through the details of her case on a website dealing with side effects of radiation like burns known as **proctitis**, I found that if this is not treated, it can develop into tumors again or the patient can lose life due to excess bleeding from the radiation burns known as **chronic radiation proctitis.**

The recommended treatment for this is a technique called APC (Argon Plasma Coagulation).

I discussed the matter with the oncologist, however, he was non-responsive, when repeatedly asked for an answer, he referred my wife to the gastroenterologist for a sigmoidoscopy, and she told it is due to radiation and advised to do APC procedure.

However, what she did during the sigmoidoscopy is very intriguing and need scrutiny. She removed a few sample pieces from the already burnt tissues i.e. radiation proctitis tissues and sent for biopsy, to ascertain whether there is any cancerous growth. This issue has angered the oncologist and he scolded the gastroenterologist for collecting the sample for biopsy without his permission.

Because of this, my wife started bleeding and has to be admitted in emergency for treatment. Though the blood count was good, due to sudden fall in platelets they administered injections to stop the bleeding.

After completion of the 2nd day of fourth cycle of chemotherapy, they discharged her from hospital.

Very Important Note

However, things were not going as expected and my wife has to face excess bleeding from the rectum again.

What happened was a very serious matter and my wife on the 2nd day after completion of the fourth cycle of chemotherapy. She developed extremely excess bleeding and in half an hour, she collapsed. Almost two bed linens were soaked in blood and she had to be shifted to the hospital.

However on the way to hospital, she regained consciousness. When admitted to the hospital emergency, her TLC and platelet count was very low. This was on July 19, 2011. However, luckily after administering several sachets of blood and platelets, the bleeding stopped.

Because of this incident, the APC procedure did not take place. Fortunately, since the APC procedure was not done. Without any further treatment, it healed on its own in about 8-9 months.

The doctor could have told us that there was no need for any special treatment for the same and it may heal on its own. Then I would not have requested him to proceed with the APC.

Once the bleeding was controlled, she was shifted to the room and she felt fine. However, on the next day around 6 am she started bleeding non-stop again and when told the oncologist, he advised some injections to prevent the bleeding and simultaneous blood and platelet transfusion. It continued until evening around 6 pm, but the bleeding did not stop at all.

Then I got angry and told the physician about her condition, though it was one of the best corporate hospital, it took another hour to shift her to an MICU. Even after shifting her to the Oncology MICU, her condition did not improve and called for fresh blood and platelet transfusion.

At this point, I felt extremely helpless and all our source of donors exhausted. Though the hospital was in a position to supply blood and platelets, the blood bank in charge doctor told me it will not be of any help as the stored platelets will not help for more than 24 hours and you have to arrange fresh platelet donors.

I prayed to god and simultaneously started searching the web sites for blood and platelets donors. Fortunately, I contacted Computer Associates, Microsoft, Google and also an old friend of mine working in Templeton office. To my utter surprise, I was flooded with offers from all the three, except Microsoft. They were very arrogant and did not care a hoot for my request, but God was with me. I have received more than enough help from CA, Google and Templeton office in Hyderabad, India.

Therefore, under such circumstances there are some important aspects, which need your attention. You need lot of blood transfusions to replenish blood loss and fresh platelet (not stored in the blood bank) replacement to stop the bleeding.

It is always better to have own blood donors like family members with the same blood group or relatives with the same blood group.

In case people in your immediate circle are not available, look for donors, especially young people in the 25-35 age group, though up to the age 50, people can donate blood and platelet, it is better to get youngsters.

Alternatively, look for volunteer blood donors in your locality, you can look for their web sites **www.AmericasBlooddonors.org** in the North America, **www.redcross.org** , **www.mybloodcenter.org** etc in US. In India there is one such web site, namely, **www.friends4support.org** Just do local web searches and you can find volunteer blood donors in your locality.

In some cases, it is difficult to find such donor web sites, such a case, contact multinational corporations like the CA (Computer Associates), Templeton, Google or any such entities in your locality.

These MNC employees donate blood almost every three-four months to blood banks. You don't know when you need blood and platelets in case the patient's condition is worst or they are categorized as Stage-III or Stage-IV.

In case of Stage IV patients, though there are some exceptions, it is extremely difficult to control the spread of cell mutation, let alone cure.

Therefore, blood and platelet donation is very essential and if help did not come at the right time, things can go out of control.

Another important aspect to remember is, if affordable, look for centers providing specialized palliative care, maybe in the hospital or may be in other places like a palliative care center located outside the hospital. Patients categorized as Stage IV, their survival rate is extremely low.

Therefore, proper care, and showing empathy with them by caring for their little requests can do great wonders . This is very crucial in the last few months of their life, especially, if the doctor said that he do not have anything else to offer.

In the MICU everyone was on their heels even after giving about 48 sachets of blood and equal number of platelets, the bleeding did not stop, ultimately on the third day after providing fresh platelets of about three sachets, i.e. 350 ml x 3, the bleeding started to stop and my wife's condition slightly improved.

Owing to excessive bleeding, her condition was almost hopeless and the doctors wanted to shift her to an isolation room fearing infection due to non-stop bleeding.

However, since my wife was conscious at that movement and wanted to get well at any cost, she told the ICU in charge doctor not to shift her to the isolation room.

Things improved fast and on the 9th day in the MICU, she recovered well and the doctor told he is stopping all medication including the remaining 2 cycles of chemotherapy. He also said this is something like a miracle.

After discharge from MICU she was advised to take rest for a month and return for further follow up. After one month, the CEA level was about 4.5, which is within the permissible limit.

The doctor advised my wife to take some oral medicines and review after three month's stay at home.

After the first three months recess, my wife's condition was better and she was as normal as anyone but with slight tiredness. Otherwise, OK. During this period, a whole abdominal Ultrasound scan, CBC, liver function test, etc. were done and found to be normal.

However, during the next visit to the doctor after another three months stay at home, i.e. on the sixth month after discharge from MICU on July 27, 2011, unfortunately in the intervening period, I did not check the CEA level in the blood since the doctor told me not to test the same very frequently.

Please note that this was again a grave mistake I did as well as the physician advised, because testing the level of CEA gives an idea whether the disease is in control or not.

In my wife's case, immediately following the visit to the doctor on the sixth month i.e. sometime in November 2011, suddenly, she felt severe pain on her back and neck. The doctor prescribed some painkillers and the routine medicines, multi vitamins, protein powder etc., and told to continue the same until the next visit after another three months.

Unfortunately, her pain did not stop and she started feeling more and more uncomfortable, especially due to the pain on her neck.

At this point the doctor advised an X-ray of the neck and followed it with a whole body bone scan. The bone scan showed normal result and the doctor said nothing to worry and come after three months for routine review.

However, within one month i.e. in early January 2012, suddenly she lost mobility. Then I have to take her to the surgical oncologist instead of the medical oncologist, as I did not feel happy about the radiologist's advice.

The surgical oncologist immediately called for a team of neurologist and on the neuro-surgeon's advice, we did an MRI scan.

The MRI scan revealed that her 5, 6 and 7 vertebrates are severely affected with cervical spine metastasis and need immediate radiation therapy on the 7th vertebra and the CEA level was also going up.

It is, therefore, very important to point out that either the bone scan technician did not do her job well, or the oncologist miss-judged the gravity of the case. In either case, the patient has to suffer and pay a heavy price for the mistake of the doctor.

Instead of the bone scan, he could have advised a whole body PET-CT scan with contrast, which will give the exact condition of the patient i.e. main status of the patient's illness.

On January 21, 2012, she became immovable and in that conditions another 17 days of radiation @ 250 cGy/fr a day was given and after that she was better.

However, the happiness did not last long, on routine blood test after a rest of one month, the CEA level was again going up and at that point it was 55 i.e. back to square one.

Immediately a whole body PET-CT scan with contrast was done and it gave very disturbing results. She developed multiple metastases in liver, lungs, nodal, throat, and cervical spine. Here is an image of her PET-CT scan report, clearly showing the metastases (secondary tumors).

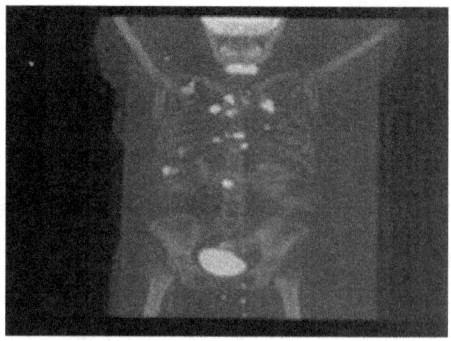

All hope of a recovery dashed at that time and my wife Prasanna asked me, Ravi is there any hope at all that she will survive and if so, how long?

I did not have an immediate answer to her question, however, I assured her that not all hope is lost and we can try whatever treatment is available.

The surgeon handed over the case to the oncologist again as he was the right person to handle the situation.

At this point, the medical oncologist-cum-radiologist, felt sorry for whatever has happened to her and done a through scrutiny of the case history to take remedial measures.

However, by this time my wife's condition was deteriorating since the CEA level has been going up and up every month i.e. from 55 to 70, then to 97, then to 128 and like that without any sign of a decrease.

During the review, they found that when the K-RAS gene mutation test done about a year ago had showed **that she had a 20% wild mutation,** but they ignored it, though I had specifically pointed out about this.

That point of time the doctor told me that since her K-RAS gene mutation was negative, i.e. NO MUTATION, there was no need to add any additional medicine to control the wild mutation. He advised another 8 cycles (weekly) of chemotherapy using Irinotecan along with 5FU, Leucovorin and in addition the use of Cetuximab (Erbitux) 400 mg as a targeted therapy.

After the chemotherapy is completed, an injection (Nupogen) will be given for three to four days for maintaining the TLC (*Total leucocyte count)* and platelet level in the body for maintaining immunity.

Irinotecan

Irinotecan, a chemotherapy drug, similar to Oxaliplatin, is used along with other chemo medicines, especially when there are secondary tumor i.e. metastases. However, it will not suit all patients and will have extreme side effect.

The main one is excessive diarrhea (loose motion). In my wife's case, though medicines were given for controlling the diarrhea, she had excessive loose motion, which will make the patient very weak.

Owing to the use of Irinotecan in the chemotherapy (second time, palliative chemotherapy between June and August 2012) made her sicker, due to excessive loose motion, resulting in bacterial infection, for which she had to undergo treatment using high dose of antibiotics.

Not once, but twice in the gap of about a month, she has to be admitted to hospital for the bacterial infection i.e. E. coli infection.

Side effects of Irinotecan

Diarrhea, nausea and vomiting, running nose, increased saliva, excess tears in the eyes, sweating, flushing, abdominal cramps, loss of appetite, feeling weak are some of the main side effects of taking Irinotecan chemo medicine.

Like any other chemo medicines, this can also lower your white blood cells count, with increased risk of infection.

Once she became normal after about two fortnight's antibiotic treatment for bacterial infection, she continued to get the palliative chemotherapy replacing Irinotecan with Oxaliplatin and Xeloda (Capacitabine) 500 mg x 2 tablets.

However, there was no improvement in her condition or any decrease in the CEA level. When asked about this, the doctor told me that CEA level is only one factor and need not bother much about it. At this point, her CEA level was 163.

However, in my personal opinion, monitoring CEA level in blood in respect of Rectal or Colon cancer, gives you an indication whether the disease is progressing or not. An increase in CEA level indicates that the disease is spreading. However, ensure that the patient did not know this information as much as possible. I.e. the increase in CEA level, because, if the patient is mentally not strong, it can affect his/her condition.

The Cetuximab (brand name Erbitux from Merk) a patented drug, is a very dangerous and exorbitantly priced medicine.

The irony is that this medicine did not give any worthwhile results in controlling the increasing CEA level or increase in Survival Rate.

Even after giving eight doses of Erbitux (Cetuximab), each having 400 mg/day, my wife did not get any benefit at all, except during first dosage, a slight i.e. a few units reduction in CEA level, but subsequently, no benefit whatsoever at all.

When questioned the manufacturer, the reply from them was that we would not answer patient queries, instead advised to tell the oncologist to contact them.

When I confronted the doctor, he told that this medicine is not giving any result in spite of giving eight dozes i.e. 8 cycles, two days medication with a gap of 7 days in between.

The oncologist told me that one medicine Avastin (Bevacizumab Injection), a patented drug, from Roche is there and he will try with it as a last resort and it was more dangerous than the Cetuximab, and costs Rs.210000 i.e. about US $ 4500 each dose of 500 mg/day.

Like the other costly medicine, this one also did not give any positive results or help increase the overall Survival Rate.

At that time I checked the history of these two medicines (both patented and monopoly drugs) from Merk and Roche respectively.

I found that the results of the drug trial has given very poor results with a maximum benefit of 4.2 to 6.5 months median benefit, to some patients, i.e. without having any worthwhile benefit of increased Survival Rate. The US FDA has withdrawn the approval for Avastin from using it for advanced Breast Cancer.

I recollect an incident that happened a year back while a friend of mine, who gave fresh platelet for my wife, told me that his father, aged about 69 years, diagnosed with advanced stage of cancer and his oncologist told him to undergo a surgery and subsequent chemotherapy and radiation.

However, after careful consideration of all facts including, cost of treatment, the age of the patient and the expected benefits vis-à-vis the side effects, if any, they decided not to proceed with the doctor's advice and let his father live as long as he may live, because of the expected troubles and side effects of the treatment.

He told me that the main reason for not proceeding with the treatment was due to his father's age. His father lived happily and passed away after six months.

Therefore, it is worthwhile to do a thorough analysis of the cost, benefits and condition of the patient including age and then take a decision about proceeding with surgery, chemotherapy, radiation therapy etc. especially if the patient is very old, and the disease was detected at an advanced stage e.g. stage III or stage IV.

Since many of the so-called-patented life saving drugs like Cetuximab (Erbitux), Avastin (Bevacizumab) etc., all these medicines priced exorbitantly high, may not be of any use, as the expected benefits are almost Zero.

In addition, the patient need not suffer from the side effects of these dangerous medicines. However, if diagnosed at an early stage, trying with these medicines, if recommended by the Oncologist, may be of help, otherwise, in the advanced stages, it is futile.

After giving three doses of Avastin, the doctor told my wife and me, now there is nothing leftover in this world for him to offer. In effect, he was telling in simple terms that look my friend, now god only can help you and prayed for the better.

This incident was on September 23, 2012. He prescribed some painkillers, multi vitamins, and the high protein drink and recommended to contact a particular pain management expert, who advised us to take Morphine based pain relievers, as it gives better results.

5 Diet Plan for Colorectal Cancer Patients

Most patients undergo chemotherapy and radiation, in addition to several other drugs during and after treatment. Therefore, it is essential to maintain proper health by taking a balanced diet. Since there are several side effects of the treatment, one should avoid certain foods and include more nutritious items in their diet. Here is a small list for your information and guidance.

Avoid

Red meat, junk (fast) foods, saturated fats, items like ice cream, ghee, pickles, refined sugar, coffee, and alcohol. Instead of tea, may use green tea.

Include More

Fruits of all varieties including grapes, apple, cranberries, blueberries etc. You can take seven to eight courses of these items daily.

However, avoid citrus fruits, if you have liver metastasis in addition, banana if you have high level of potassium in the blood or diabetic.

Include lot of vegetables; like spinach and other leafy vegetables, cauliflower, cabbage, broccoli, tomato. Also use, spices like turmeric, ginger, onion, garlic, leek, and cinnamon in your daily use.

In addition, you can take dry fruits - almonds, walnut, and pistachio, say a fist full of it daily. You can also include egg white, fish - salmon, tuna, or mackerel, in moderate quantity in your diet.

6 The Crucial Last Stage of the Patient

When in December 2012, my wife Prasanna was admitted to the hospital due to total loss of mobility, by that time the disease had spread to all parts of the body (metastasis i.e. secondary tumors spread from the primary tumor) through the already positive lymph nodes, prior to surgery or during the radiation therapy. She had multiple metastases in the liver, lungs, nodal, throat, and cervical spine.

Since the metastases spread to the spine from neck to vertebrae 7,6,5, she had extreme pain on the back, shoulders and the entire body. In spite of giving, her narcotic pain relievers, she did not get any relief from the pain.

Pain management will be an important aspect of treatment post doctor's expression of inability to do any further treatment i.e. Stage-IV medication in addition to need for palliative care.

The morphine-based painkillers were more effective in my wife's case as it reduced the pain on the bones like spine, shoulder etc.

The main side effect of using Morphine or such other narcotic based pain killers is the severe vomiting. However, vomiting can be controlled with medicines.

Palliative Care

Once the doctor said that he/she is helpless, there is no hope, except pray to god for alms or miracles. Therefore, in the last stages of the patient, i.e. the last few months, proper care and mental support is very essential, because the patients movements will be limited, mostly bed ridden, unable to take proper food, even if taken, feeling no taste because of the chemotherapy and other medicines including the narcotic pain relievers.

The Last One Month

I believe, this is the most crucial period of the life a colon/rectal cancer patient, for that matter of any type of cancer, irrespective of the name or location of the tumor. The patient will be in her/his most vulnerable condition with severe pain, excessive heat due to the multiplication of cells (i.e. gene mutation) taking place in the body. Mostly bed ridden, vomiting, diarrhea, sleeplessness, and all kinds of other difficulties are there.

Therefore, it is very essential to have someone by the side of the patient always, irrespective of day or night, to provide whatever small help and mental support i.e. pacifying the patient. This gesture will make the patient more comfortable.

After the doctor expressed helplessness in providing any further treatment as there is none available, we prayed to god for mercy.

From September 23, 2012, a few of my Christian friends, who are believers in prayer and provide voluntary prayer service to patients especially Cancer patients came home and prayed almost every fortnight till January 9, 2013 on which day she breathed her last.

During the intervening period from September 23, 2012 through January 9, 2013 my wife Prasanna had many strange things happening to her. Some of them are as follows:

During many of the days she felt that she is seeing a small insect (Fire Fly) with its rear lights on, sitting on a corner of the bedroom door looking at her. She told me about this on several times, but when I check at that spot, I could not find anything at all. However, she used tell me even thereafter that the insect (Fire Fly) is looking at her and flying from one corner to another in the room.

Another incident that used to take place in her last days are, on a few occasions, she used to talk to her mother, as if her mother is sitting there on the bedroom corner, and tell, mummy please feed me I feel hungry and for many days I have not eaten anything.

One day, evening (almost 8 pm), my wife Prasanna told me that her mother fed her well and it was very tasty food. These things seem strange, may be true, because the patient may be feeling so.

On another day, one more strange thing happened.(this was in the last week of December 2012) In the night, Prasanna cried out and told me that she saw many strange human like creatures both men and women, looks like demons, were trying to pull her up. I feel this again, is a sign of things to come in future and indicates that her life is nearing to an end.

However, this particular incident happened just ten days before she passed away is extremely surprising and sad to note.

She told me in the morning that she saw a dream in the early morning and felt that as if she was dead and lying on the floor of the front room of our house. Hearing this I felt that this is a clear indication of nearing her end. This was exactly ten days before her last breath.

Some other indications that were giving signals of her end is very near was that she stopped taking food, except some milk, tea or water. No solid foods. She did not have any hunger, but extreme pain especially on her neck, spine, and skeletal system like shoulders.

This was due to the spread of metastases to liver, nodal, thorax, neck, cervical spine and to several vertebrae. In addition, she had loose motion, not passing of stool continuously for at a stretch of 7 to 8 days and was unable to walk even 10-15 feet from the bed.

Again, especially at night time, she felt extremely uncontrollable urge for dying, because of the pain and excessive heat in her body. In addition, she no longer wanted to live. That was the mental condition due to extreme stress.

Just about three days ago, i.e. on January 7, she told me Ravi don't go anywhere, be with me I may not last much and I feel that I am sinking. So I did not go anywhere, I also felt that her days are nearing to an end. I want to do whatever possible for her. My daughter, who was a medical student, was also with us.

On the fateful day i.e. on January 9, 2013 in the midnight, she showed me her hands and told it is freezing, when I touched her hands, I also felt the cold freezing sensation. This was again an indication of her losing vital parameters. Immediately I checked her pulse and BP, the pulse rate was very high and the BP almost 168, indicating the high-risk levels.

Since the doctor expressed his inability three months ago, we decided not to go to the hospital and face whatever is going to happen with great mental strength and control of emotions.

At around 4 am on January 9, 2013, she asked for some sweets, but we did not had any sweets at home. Instead of sweets, I told her that tea is there and I will prepare and give.

She readily agreed and I prepared some tea with sugar and gave her. She, like a small child, drank the tea and nodded her head in satisfaction.

An hour later around 5 am, she murmured that I (Ravi) didn't come from office and called my daughter. Then I told her that my daughter just now only slept I will call her later on. She again agreed with me and tried to sleep.

The Last Breath

On January 9, 2013 at around 7.42 am, she asked me to call my daughter and take her to the bathroom. After passing urine, we brought her to the bed.

While trying to sit on the bed, I felt that she just jerked and her body became very loose. My daughter and me were still holding her and trying to make her sit on the bed and make her comfortable.

However, in just a few seconds later while she was in our hands she breathed her last at exactly at 07.45 am on January 9, 2013. In spite of all the efforts and sufferings, the end came unexpectedly.

When all hopes were lost, the Pentecostal Christian friends prayer offer, we felt she may get some relief and Jesus may provide her another life. However, in spite of prayers by several brothers and sisters, there was no change in her condition and things were going from bad to worst. I even requested the Joyce Myer prayer group to pray for my wife, which they did.

A sister who claims as a cancer specialist in prayers, had offered a solution - a prayer extending thirty days including a fasting prayer for 21 days. However, she was not charging us any money,   i.e. it was a charity offer. She used to call up us in the early morning around 5 am and prayed for my wife's recovery exactly for 30 days. On her advice, I even destroyed the idols of some gods, kept at my home for daily worship, thinking that these idols may be blocking her recovery.

There was no improvement in my wife's condition. I again contacted another brother, who is more popular in offering prayers for the recovery of patients. With great difficulty, I located this brother and requested him to pray for my wife's recovery.

He prayed for two days and promised to call us every day early morning until she recovers from her disease. However, there was no need for him to call us the next day, because, in the early morning on January 9, 2013 at 07.45 am, my wife Prasanna passed away.

Therefore, what lesson I learnt from this incident is that when medicines and treatments cannot improve anything at all, the prayers or expectations of a miracle may be a myth. There may be exceptions and miracles might have happened but it is very rare. At the time of birth itself, your fate is written by the almighty. No one can change the fate, not even any God.

Recommended reading for enriching your knowledge, the following web sites are of immense help to patients as well as their immediate relatives, friends and people who are curious to know detailed information about various types of cancer, its diagnosis, and treatment. They are:

www.cancer.org, promoted by American Cancer Society, **www.cancerresearchuk.org** promoted by Cancer Research Society, UK.

There are several other web sites built by voluntary organizations as well as highly reputed hospitals. Just searching the web, you can find several useful sites.

In like USA, there are strict adherence to regulations and medical treatments by doctors. However, in countries like India, there is very little scope for fighting mistakes by medical professionals as people did not have the resources to fight them due to inordinate delays in court cases and grant of very little compensation.

I, therefore, strongly suggest, if you think that there is extreme and willful neglect by the medical professionals, i.e. oncologists both surgeon and physicians, do not hesitate to take legal remedies for mitigation of grievances.

7 Alternate Therapy

I, recently, came across in some cancer forums about use of alternate therapy (in place of surgery, chemo, and radiation) for treating different types of cancers.

They use highly concentrated form of Hemp Oil aka, Cannabis Oil, i.e 95% and above (extracted from Marijuana, a banned narcotic), which many people claims to have given very positive results.

The production and sale of such drugs is prohibited in the US and elsewhere. However, there is mention about the efficacy of this drug on the web site of **www.cancer.gov.** Even some States in the USA has given permission to produce the Cannabis Oil at home for medicinal purpose.

You may read the complete article including precautions, side effects, etc on their site. Please copy and paste the following web address on to your browser to read

http://www.cancer.gov/cancertopics/pdq/cam/cannabis/ healthprofessional/page1/AllPages

I Hope this short essay enlightens you and if satisfied, please spread the word about this Book amongst your circle of friends, relatives and colleagues or whatever media you can.

REQUEST

If possible, please write an honest review and rate it. The customer review option is available just below the book cover on Amazon listing page.

I will donate the entire proceeds from the sale of this Book to poor and needy cancer patients.

www.ingramcontent.com/pod-product-compliance
Lightning Source LLC
Chambersburg PA
CBHW071755170526
45167CB00003B/1038